FOREWORD

I am both delighted and privileged to be endorsing this book. Before being introduced to David Hogg, I had put him in that box where all the other fitness experts I'd ever met, were. My experience had been of being pushed too hard, too quickly and as a result losing my motivation for the gym with its big, horrible machines. David's approach is so different and this book is a testament to the personal and easy manner that he promotes exercise and wellbeing.

Exercise does not have to mean wearing lycra, pumping iron and having loud music play in the background. It is recommended that walking 10,000 steps a day will significantly improve your health and wellbeing and with that reduce the risk of cancer and heart disease. However, it is hard to do, especially when you get older and can feel less confident whilst on your feet. Seated exercise is an excellent opportunity to build confidence and keep your muscles supple and this book not only talks about, but shows you exactly how to do these exercises.

Earlier this year, David was short listed for an ITV Feelgood Factor Award for Pride of Britain. This did not only honour his commitment to helping people live healthier lives, but also his ability to reach out and support people of any age, from any background. Although he didn't win, I feel that the personal journey David has made in writing this book, is worth more than a shiny award. Health and wellbeing is not a quick fix and David's journey is proof that good things come to those that wait. Enjoy!!

Alison Cowie
Director of Public Health
NHS West Essex
October 2009

ACTIVE HEALTH
50 PLUS

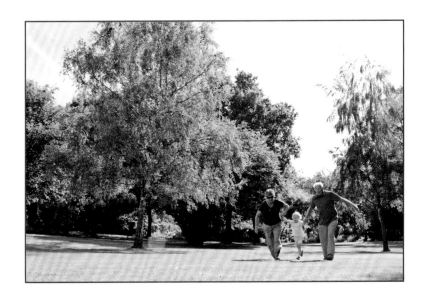

In memory of Pamela Hogg
4th October 1947 – 17th October 2005

DAVID HOGG

DOCTORS' ENDORSEMENTS

'Physical activity and exercise carry the burden of major misconceptions. Society associates these terms with youth, vigour and perfect health. Thus, it can easily be considered as unsuitable or even dangerous for the physically less able. The cause for limited physical activity is often multi-factorial. Chronic illness, disability, obesity, mental health problems, age and many other issues can act as perceived barriers.'

'Exercise is also linked to endurance, exhaustion and pain. None of this has to be true if good physical and emotional health, rather than competitive achievement, is the target'.

'Physical activity can be as simple, easy and pleasurable as desired and still be effective if main-tained and incorporated into our daily lives. Strength to climb the stairs in our home, flexibility to tie our shoelaces, endurance to complete our shopping, etc., can be worthwhile goals to work towards. Many of my patients worry mostly about the potential loss of their independence. A regular adherence to a low impact activity programme, as introduced by David Hogg could achieve this worthwhile target.'

'David Hogg has a formidable understanding of these intrapersonal barriers. His approachable personality, fine sense of humour and professionalism have helped many of my patients to find a pleasurable way back into physical activity- and maintain their interest.'

Dr Saadet Lauble

MRCGP DFFP DRCOG MSc Sport & Exercise Medicine

'Keeping physically fit is an important factor in achieving a sense of well-being and indeed of being physically and mentally well. Well-trained muscles are much less likely to suffer pains and strains and a well-trained body is likely to help keep one's mind happy. The importance of mod-erate and vigorous exercise in the treatment of mild and even moderate depression has been documented in clinical trails.

This book provides an introduction to simple exercises that can easily slot into one's daily routine. It is written with safety in mind and quite rightly emphasises gradual increase in the length and strenuousness of any exercise programme. It is easy to read and an excellent guide to anybody who wants to start and maintain an exercise programme for healthier body and mind.'

Dr. J.M. Pechan – Chigwell Medical Centre

ACTIVE HEALTH 50 PLUS

SECTION 1 - ACTIVE HEALTH

SECTION 2 - SEATED EXERCISES

THOUGHTS FROM THE AUTHOR

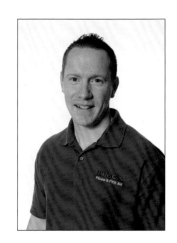

Throughout my career, I have been passionate about helping people of all ages to improve their lives through health, fitness and social interaction. This passion has enabled me to meet hundreds of new people whom I have trained through exercise, teaching them the vast benefits of leading a physically active and socially fulfilling life. Many have become lifelong friends.

I have always been an active person - whether fitness training, taking part in sport or even cleaning my car vigorously - and the benefits I have found from this have been amazing.

At school I found that I did well at most sports but academically, I tended to really struggle. Leaving school with below average grades, I continued to have difficulties with reading and writing, but I developed a number of my own strategies to overcome this with the support of my parents, who taught me the true values in life.

My first job was at a local sports centre, where I met Gary O'Connor, the Centre's Health and Fitness Manager. Gary was a huge and positive influence on me over the years we worked together and we are still very good friends. He taught me about the importance of health and fitness for the body and mind, and that it doesn't have to hurt to do you good!

As my career in leisure and health developed, I decided to see a hypnotherapist to help with my fears and insecurities, and Diana Powley from Dune Hypnotherapy was recommended to me. I soon found that Diana has an amazing gift. She immediately suggested ways that I could help improve my reading and writing and she gave me the confidence to address my fears. Soon after seeing Diana, I was encouraged to have a dyslexia test and was diagnosed as being severely dyslexic. Knowing this gave me immense confidence, as for years I had thought my problems were somehow down to me being careless or lazy.

To say that I have been lucky to work with so many great and supportive people and have such a wonderful family would be an understatement. I would love to mention them all, but may save that for my autobiography!

I have always wanted to write a book to enable me to pass on some of the great life-changing experience that I have accumulated over the years and I have decided to dedicate this, my first book, to my Mum, who we sadly lost to cancer in 2005. Mum's death was very unexpected and I clearly remember the night before her funeral, when I sat down at the computer and wrote her a letter saying how grateful I was to have such a loving Mum. I also promised her that I would always strive to be the best I could and never let anything get in the way of achieving my dreams.

I therefore hope that you will use the ideas in this book to improve your own enjoyment of life and maybe reach some of your dreams and aspirations, through gaining better health and well-being.

David hogg

SAFETY ADVICE ON ACTIVE HEALTH

Before you embark on your new lifestyle, there are a few Health & Safety things that you need to consider ......

1. If you are new to exercise or adapting your eating habits, it is important that you arrange to see your GP first, just to make sure that he/she is happy for you to commence your new lifestyle change. It will be useful to take this book along with you, so that your Doctor can see the level of exertion and type of things that you will be trying.

2. When you start exercising, there is one key thing that you must do – **BREATHE!** For some strange reason, every time I take a Seated Exercise class everyone wants to hold their breath! I think this is because they are concentrating on their technique so much that the simple things like breathing are forgotten, so please remember this one thing.

3. Another important thing to keep a check on is your posture. Try to maintain a neutral (or natural) spine by standing tall, as this will help strengthen your core muscles and reduce the risk of injury. And, when performing any type of exercise, always work to your own range of movement so that you do not compromise your correct body posture.

4. Before taking part in physical activity or exercise, always consider the environment that you are in. When you are outdoors there are a number of things to be mindful of including the weather, floor surface condition, other people, traffic, animals and insects. When you are working indoors, make sure that the room temperature is suitable. You don't want the room to be too cold or too hot. It might be a good idea to exercise in a room that has a window, to allow some natural light in and so that it can be opened if you begin to feel too hot. You also need to position yourself in an area that gives you enough space to perform the activity you are going to take part in!

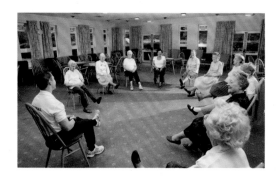
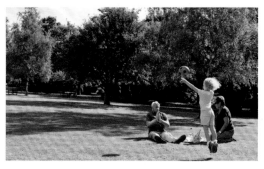

WHAT IS YOUR CURRENT STATE OF HEALTH?

The following questionnaire will help you to check whether you are ready to start the exercises in this book. If you answer **'YES' to any of the questions,** or have doubts about your suitability to exercise, **you must consult your doctor before doing so!!**

PLEASE TICK	YES	NO
Do you have heart disease or any other cardiovascular, respiratory or blood pressure problems?		
Is there history of heart disease in your family?		
Do you ever have pain in your heart or chest?		
Do you often get headaches, or feel faint or dizzy?		
Do you suffer from pain or limited movement in any joints, which has been caused by exercise or may be aggravated by exercise?		
Are you taking any drugs or medication at the moment, or, recuperating from a recent illness or operation?		
Do you have any other medical condition, which you may think may affect your ability to exercise, such as asthma or diabetes?		

If you answered **'NO' to all the questions,** this is a reasonable assurance that it is safe for you to start exercising – but you may want to speak to your GP to be sure.

EXERCISE GUIDELINES

Don't forget that you should always speak to your GP before starting an exercise programme.

- Never exercise if you feel tired, unwell or after eating a meal.
- Ensure that you wear loose, comfortable clothing and footwear (no heeled shoes!) well-fitting slippers/trainers are ideal.
- Always begin with good posture (straight back and stand up 'tall') and keep a check on it.
- Never hold your breath during exercises.
- Warm up first and do the exercises at your own pace and level of ability.

If you experience pain, feel dizzy or unwell, slowly stop exercising and consult your doctor. It is important to take your time and build up your exercise programme gradually. Any exercise programme should be a pleasure, not a pain. Remember to keep drinking water throughout your exercise programme to replace any water you have lost.

Exercise should be gradual, comfortable and frequent (20-30 minutes 3-5 times a week) and **most of all enjoyable.**

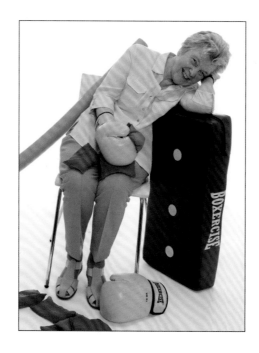

BALANCE PROBLEMS

Balance disorders can be difficult to diagnose, because it is hard to describe their symptoms to a doctor. You may use words such as "dizzy", "woozy" or "light headed", to describe what you are feeling. For some people, the feeling can be brief, whilst for others it can last a long time, disrupting their daily lives.

If you do experience any 'balance' problems please don't ignore them, as they could be serious. Sometimes they are a sign of other health problems, such as those affecting the brain, the heart, or circulation of the blood. They are also a particular cause of falls and fall-related injuries in older people. For these reasons, it is important to have a balance disorder diagnosed and treated as soon as possible.

Ask yourself the following questions. *If you answer "yes" to any of these questions, you should discuss the symptom with your doctor!*

- Do I feel unsteady?
- Do I feel as if the room is 'spinning' or moving around me?
- Do I feel as if I'm moving when I know I'm standing or sitting still?
- Do I lose my balance completely and fall?
- Do I feel as if I'm falling?
- Do I feel "light headed" or as if I might faint?
- Does my vision become blurred?
- Do I ever feel disoriented, losing my sense of time, place, or identity?

If you think that you have a balance disorder, you should schedule an appointment with your doctor as soon as possible and let your doctor know all your symptoms.

Things that may help improve your balance:

- Use a walking aid when you are out and about!
- Take your shoes to the shoe mender's and have him put a thin rubber sole on them with a good grip.
- Work on your co-ordination skills by doing simple exercises like rotating your hand in a circular motion in one direction and then in the other direction. Then try rotating your hands in the opposite direction to one-another. Try the same with your feet (while sitting down!)
- To practice hand-to-eye co-ordination, throw and catch a sponge ball in one hand a few times, then change hands. Then throw the ball from one hand and catch it in the other.
- Get your hearing checked out, as impaired hearing can cause balance problems.

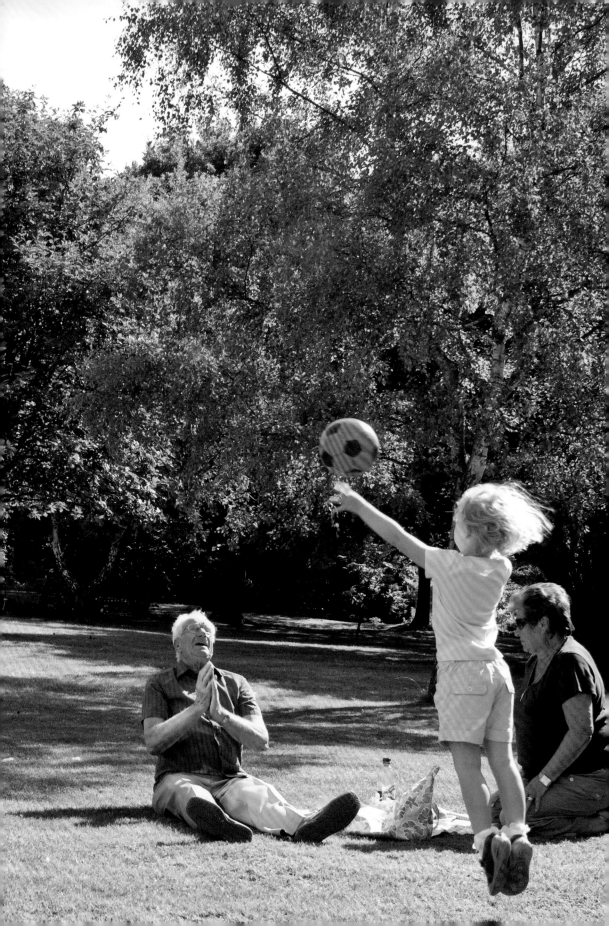

BARRIERS AND MISCONCEPTIONS AROUND PHYSICAL ACTIVITY

We all know that exercise is good for us, but not many people do enough of it because of a number of barriers or misconceptions. This is why I think it is important to highlight these before you start on any new lifestyle changes.

To most people the word exercise is quite 'scary', as it is associated with feeling pain and working hard to improve physical condition. You may also have had a 'bad experience' with exercise at some point in your life - this could be the memory of your PE lessons at school, of running around a field on a cold (possibly wet) day and then having to shower in front of everyone?

Some of the other reasons people don't take part in regular activity are:

- Being too tired to get started.
- Embarrassment and lack of confidence.
- Fear of doing too much and feeling pain in the following days.
- Medical conditions or injuries.
- Concerns that physical activity will do more harm than good.

I can understand why people feel this way, but would like to reassure you that, with the right advice and guidance, improving health and fitness can be easier than you think and very enjoyable!

In the time that I have studied health and fitness, I have helped hundreds, if not thousands, of people to improve their health and well-being and overcome their barriers towards physical activity and this has been achieved by two simple steps:

Step 1 - Introduce 'easy' daily activities such as taking the stairs instead of the lift, or getting off the bus one stop before a regular stop and then walking the rest of the way.

Step 2 - Find an activity that you think you will enjoy that involves body movement and getting slightly out of breath, that you can access at least once a week.

If you do this, in a short time your confidence will grow, your fears will reduce, energy levels will increase and your perception of physical activity will change. Before you know it, you will be trying to convert the unconverted!

SO, WHAT ARE THE BENEFITS OF PHYSICAL ACTIVITY AND KEEPING ACTIVE?

It is amazing how ageing affects the body and how quickly quality of life can be compromised when our activity levels are reduced, **but on the other side of the coin,** the lifestyle benefits of regular exercise are incredible. Exercise improves circulation, strengthens muscles and joints, and enables you to do more than before. You will find that you are able to do everyday tasks more easily and will not get so tired. You should also sleep better and find that you are more relaxed.

Regular exercise can also effectively reduce the symptoms of arthritis; it helps to control blood pressure, encourages a better posture and lowers your risk of osteoporosis - therefore helping to reduce injury from accidental falls. It helps to reduce depression and lowers the risk of heart disease and stroke and can prolong independence. The other good news is that it's **never too late** to reap the benefits of physical activity and **even very elderly muscles remain fully responsive to regular exercise!**

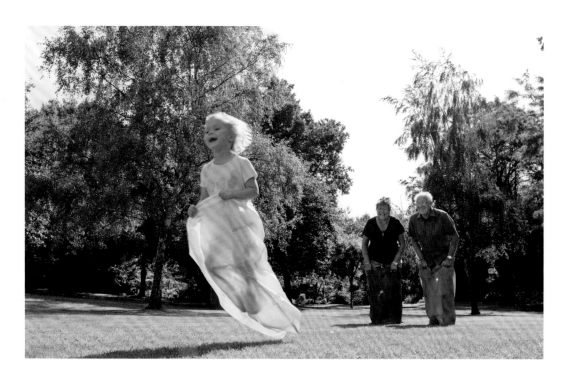

WHY WARM UP?

A warm up should always consist of mobility rotations, a 'pulse raiser' to increase the heart rate to make you feel warmer, and a short stretch. This allows the blood to flow to the working muscles and increase the fluid to the joints. It also increases the air intake to the lungs. These together prepare the body both mentally and physically for exercise.

A warm up can be performed for any type of activity. If we use gardening as an example, for some people, getting out the equipment that is needed to cut the grass and do some weeding etc., is enough to get their body temperature elevated. All that is needed then is to introduce a few mobility movements like hand, foot and shoulder rotations. Before you start cutting the grass, why not do a bit of weeding in the areas of the garden that require you to reach over or bend down? This allows you to stretch out some of those big muscles in your legs, back and shoulders.

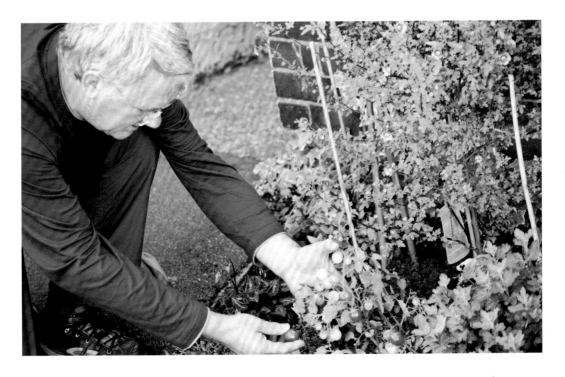

WHY DEVELOP STRENGTH?

Stimulating and strengthening your major muscles keeps them 'toned'. This makes everyday tasks a lot easier so getting out of a chair, picking something up off the floor, walking to the shops or getting out of the bath is much less of an effort. With regular strength training, the tissues surrounding the muscles become stronger and more stable, which makes the muscles more efficient at releasing their energy.

Bone density begins to decline after the age of 40, but this loss accelerates around the age of 50 years. As a result of 'bone loss', older people are more prone to bone fractures. **However,** any weight bearing exercise helps to keep bones healthy and strong!

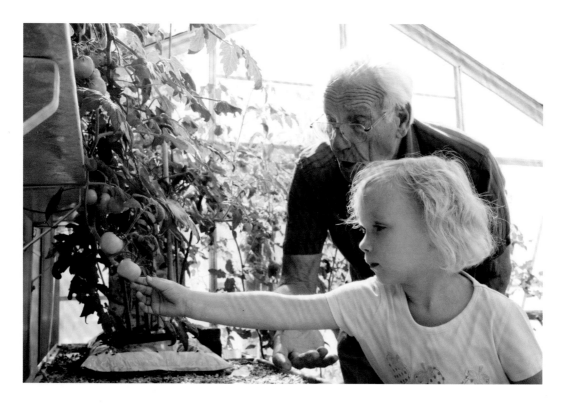

WHY DEVELOP STAMINA?

As explained previously, by stimulating muscles through exercise, they will develop and grow stronger and become more efficient at doing their job. The heart is also a muscle and with regular exercise (30 minutes of moderate to intense exercise on most days of the week) you will strengthen your heart and lungs, improve your circulation and, believe it or not, *you will feel less tired!*

As we are working the heart you will feel your heart beat quicker than normal and you will feel warmer and rosy; you should also be breathing deeper although still able to talk. Please note you should not feel faint, nauseous or struggling for breath. *If you feel pain or discomfort STOP exercising and consult your doctor.*

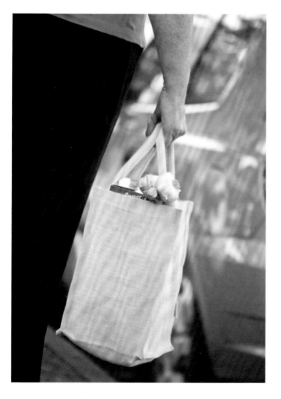
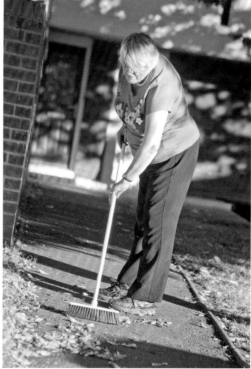

WHY COOL DOWN?

Cooling down prepares the body to stop exercising by decreasing the heart rate gradually. It helps prevent 'tenderness' after exercising and helps to maintain and develop flexibility in muscles that are tight. A good cool down will assist in the prevention of cramps, releases unnecessary tension and aids relaxation.

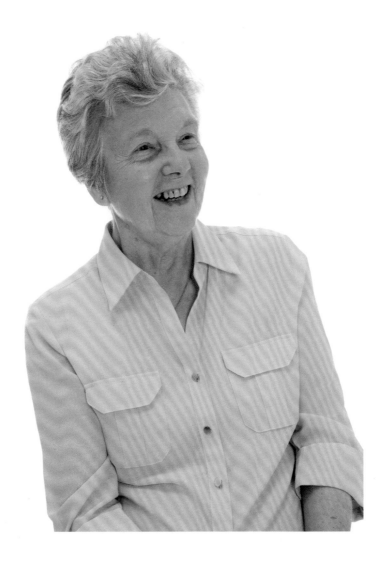

WHAT IS PHYSICAL ACTIVITY?

Physical activity is a broad term meaning any body movement that uses up energy or that causes the body to work harder than normal. *It is not just exercise and sport,* it also includes activities such as gardening, walking, hanging out your washing, carrying objects and even housework!

Physical activity is important to achieve good health and wellbeing, so I would encourage you to move as much as you can throughout the day and enjoy some 'structured' activities 2 or 3 times a week. These activities could include fitness classes, singing and dancing, exercising in the gym or organised sport. They are particularly valuable as you will be supervised by a professional person who will help you to achieve a good technique. *Don't forget that it is also a chance to meet other people with similar interests to yourself!*

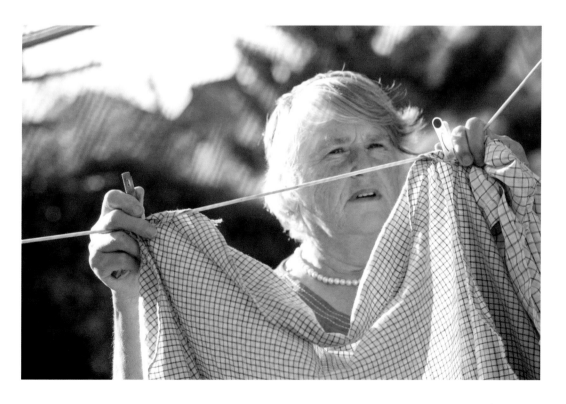

WHAT IS GOOD HEALTH?

Good health is probably the most important thing in life. Without good health we may experience debilitating disease and a poor quality of life. It is relatively easy to achieve good health, but it may involve certain changes in your lifestyle that are sometimes hard to do at first. ***The most important thing to remember is to begin slowly and to make small changes!***

Exercise helps us achieve good health by strengthening the cardiovascular system, strengthening muscles and, more importantly, reducing stress on the body. Try to find exercises that you ***enjoy*** as you will find it easier to sustain this type of activity.

Healthy eating is also very important in achieving and maintaining good health. Take notice of the frequent 'healthy eating' messages such as eating five portions of fruit and vegetables a day, drinking plenty of water (2 litres daily) and trying and eat regular meals throughout the day. The aim is to ***slowly change your eating habits for the better.***

Excessive smoking and drinking is certainly detrimental to health, but that's not to say that you need to stop drinking altogether. Mixing with people and sensible drinking can have positive effects on your emotional well-being, but remember, ***moderation is the key!***

There is no such exception for smoking! If you are a smoker, you need to go to your doctor to discuss a smoking cessation programme, as smoking endangers your health and that of others around you. ***If you stop smoking now,*** in time, your body can begin to repair any damage caused. If that's not enough motivation to make you stop, think about the money you will save!

If you have any general medical concerns as you age, visit your doctor to discuss them, as it is always better to identify these in the early stages.

Mental Health

This is something that I think is often forgotten about or overlooked. As you age, you face many changes that will affect your mental health. Your children will move away from home, people you love will die and you may retire from work. Coping with all these changes is difficult, but it can be done. You need to be able to accept your individual circumstances and stay interested in and involved with life.

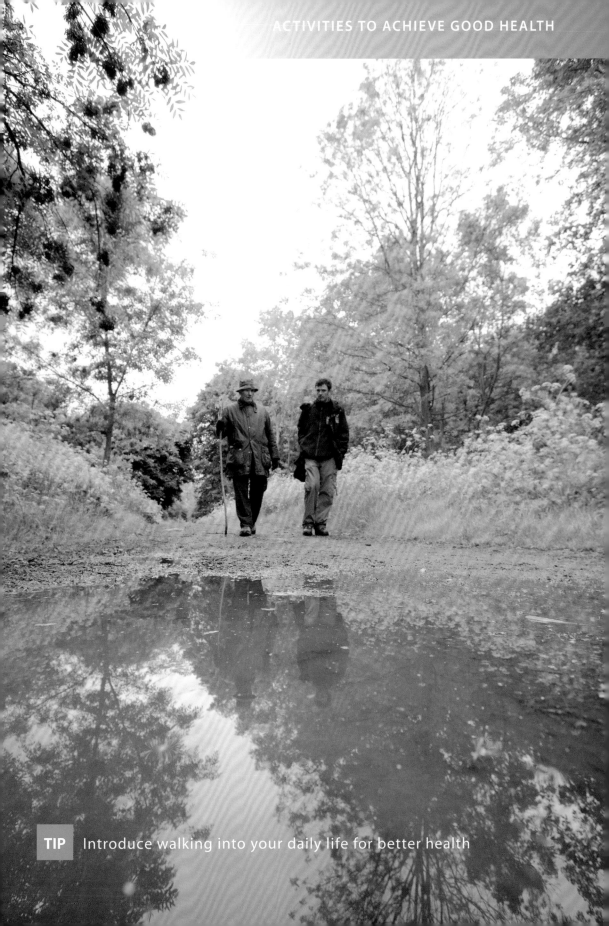

TIP Introduce walking into your daily life for better health

WALKING FOR HEALTH

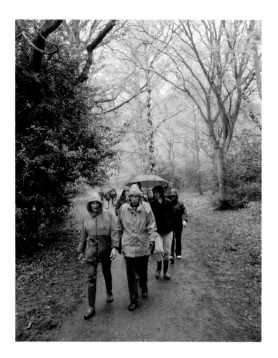

Walking is a great way to achieve good health for the simple reason that it is free and requires no specialised equipment. It is accessible to everyone regardless of age, income, where you live, or your ability. This type of activity can be done individually or as part of a group. Personally, I would always recommend walking in a group or with a friend for the social benefits and safety reasons. Walking can also easily be incorporated into your daily life. If you are interested in walking with a group, visit your local Information Centre and ask for details of walks in your area.

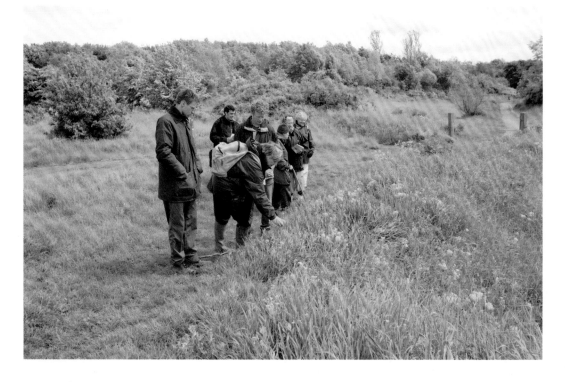

When you decide to go for a walk, try to structure it in three stages:

Stage one: Warm up - start slowly and after five minutes gradually increase your walking pace.

Stage two: Brisk walk - increase your walking pace to a level where you begin to feel warm and slightly out of breath. (Please note that this is a level where you are able to hold a conversation with someone).

Stage three: Cool down - reduce your speed to allow your breathing to reduce to its normal state, and to let your body temperature return to normal.

Route planning

When planning your walking route it is important to ensure that it is suitable for your level of fitness. You will need to consider whether you choose a route with a gradient (hill) in it and where possible, try to avoid crossing any roads.

You will also need to consider the possible hazards you may encounter on route. These can include dog walkers, cyclists, stiles, uneven floor surfaces, open water or flooded areas as well as weather conditions such as hot sunshine, high winds, heavy rain, fog or snow.

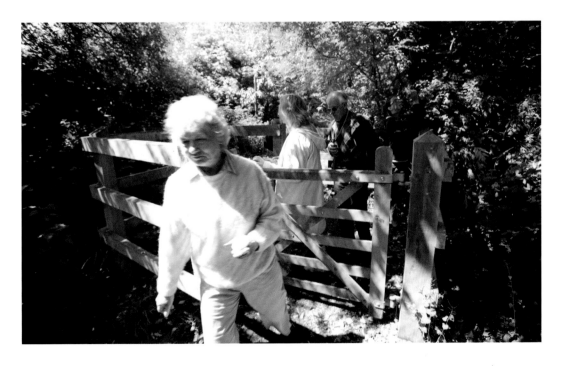

GARDENING FOR FITNESS

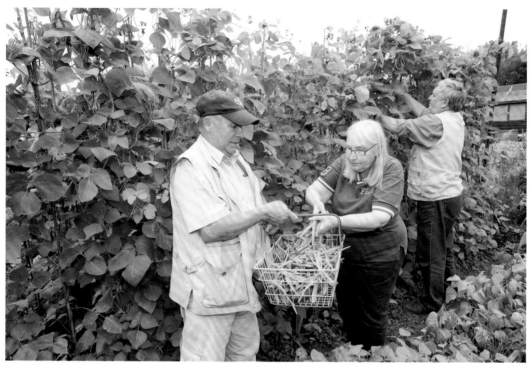

Catering for a vegatable garden provides healthy exercise and nutritional food crops

I don't claim to be an expert when it comes to gardening, but tending a garden myself, I know this type of activity has a remarkable effect on my general health.

Gardening has many health and therapeutic benefits for older people, especially if you can create an 'edible' garden. Why not grow your own organic, healthy food and turn your garden into a source of delight. Your edible garden can be grown in pots, grow bags, an old wheelbarrow, raised bed, green house or straight in the ground.

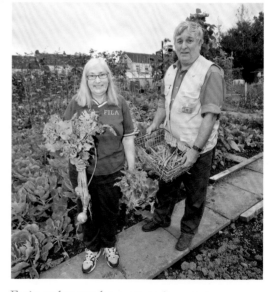

Eating what you have grown is a great satisfaction

There are many different types of activity involved in gardening and these will all challenge your fitness levels and muscles in different ways:

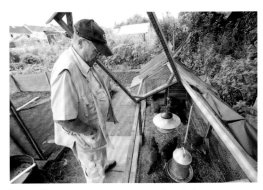

This allotments association takes it in turns to care for their chickens and enjoy the eggs produced on a shared basis

- digging
- planting
- watering
- food preparation
- harvesting
- lifting
- carrying

Finding advice about gardening is usually very easy. Why not speak to your next-door neighbours, buy a gardening magazine, talk to your local council, visit the library or join a gardening group? The list is endless. The great thing about this as part of your fitness activity is that it is really easy to do and the rewards are phenomenal!

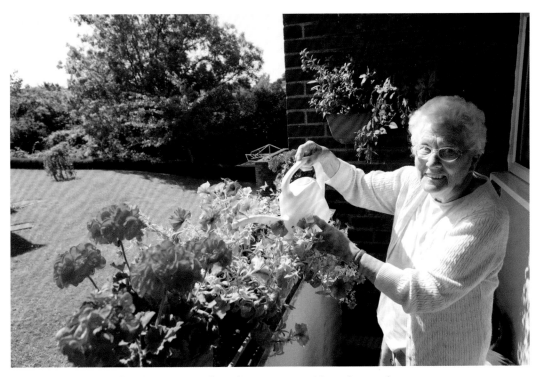

Looking after a window box or a small garden is manageable and rewarding

RELAXATION - Diana Powley SQHP

Do you enjoy walking in the countryside, or perhaps by a river, or the sea? Perhaps there is a pastime that you enjoy where you lose all sense of time when you're doing it.

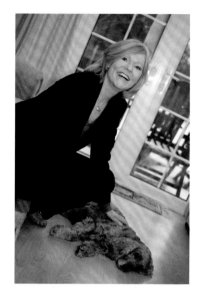

We can be physically engrossed in doing something which focuses our mind to such an extent that we switch off from all the day-to-day rush and hurry or stresses of life.

We might be sitting down with our feet up, or in bed, and imagining ourselves to be in a beautiful place – such as relaxing on a beach or in a meadow or woodland, Again we are switching off from any stress or anxieties.

Take time out each day to 'switch off', to let go of day-to-day issues. Think about what you enjoy doing. Do you play a sport or have a hobby? You might enjoy dog walking, gardening, artwork, knitting, sewing, sailing or fishing. You could lose yourself in doing what you do well, or enjoy taking up a new hobby or pastime. Do what enables you to lose yourself in something which engrosses you. Be creative.

Sometimes it can be more appropriate to physically relax. Try playing some relaxing music, putting your feet up and allowing your mind to visualise a peaceful scene. You might be picturing yourself doing what you love, or in a favourite place, or remembering a wonderful holiday. As you do this, try slowing down your breathing. This will automatically slow down your heart rate and lower your blood pressure.

All these things are calming and relaxing your whole body – every nerve, every muscle, every cell of your body is relaxed.

You are giving your nervous system a holiday, a break, the chance to heal, to rejuvenate.

Take a few moments out of your day to really relax and you will soon notice that you are generally calmer and more easy-going. Consequently you might find an improvement in your health and wellbeing, such as a lowered heart rate and blood pressure.

So take time out for you – and live a longer, healthier, happier life!

CLEAR THINKING - MIND GAMES

To help keep good mental health you can exercise your brain with crosswords, word searches, jigsaw puzzles or a range of other brain games that are available. This will help keep your memory and thinking skills 'sharp' as you age. It could even slow the development of conditions like dementia and Alzheimer's disease.

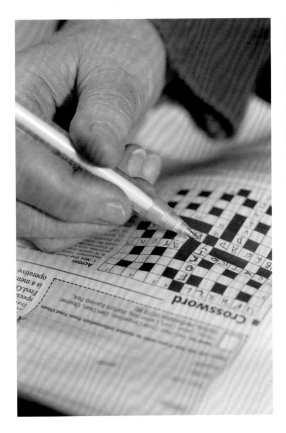

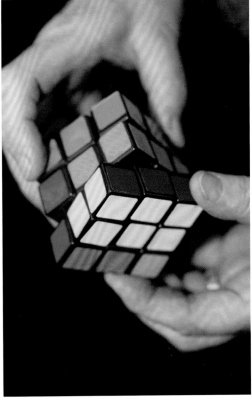

NUTRITION – (THE 'FUEL' YOU PUT IN YOUR BODY!)

In recent years, it has become almost impossible to pick up a magazine or newspaper, watch television or listen to the radio, without being confronted with articles or advice on diets. But from my experience, a lot of people are confused about what a diet is. Most people's perception of the word 'diet' is 'eating to lose weight'. However, a diet is *your regular eating lifestyle.* Lots of people think that by cutting out fat completely they will lose weight and be healthier. This is not true, as you need 'good fats' in your daily diet. Stick with Mediterranean style fats such as olive oil, fish, nuts and avocados, as these reduce the likelihood of heart disease or cancer, and have the added health benefits of lowering cholesterol and protecting your joints.

Whilst I do not endorse 'Hollywood fad' non-carbohydrate diets, it is true that many people over-eat carbohydrates - especially processed ones. Try cutting your usual portions of bread, rice, pasta or potatoes in half and substituting this with a cup of vegetables such as broccoli, cauliflower or courgettes instead. A cup of white rice contains 250 calories, whereas a cup of steamed mixed vegetables has only 50 calories. Also be aware that 'skipping meals' throughout the day **will never help shed pounds of fat.** Instead, it can lead to 'binge-eating' at night, which is a great way to pile on the pounds. Try to eat your larger meals earlier in the day and down size the portion the later it gets! Food eaten in the morning is likely to be used to supply energy during the day but calories taken in during the evening that go 'unused' end up stored as fat!

Drinking plenty of water throughout the day is essential for maintaining health and ensuring optimal mental and physical performance and can actually **help to get rid of waste products.** Water helps mobilise fat stores, while dehydration (lack of enough water) prompts fat to 'sit tight'.

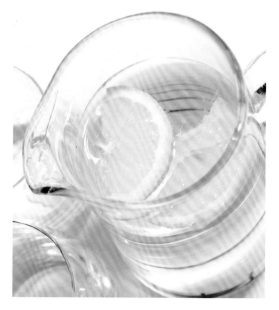

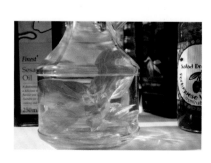

When you decide to follow a new eating plan, allow some *'cheat days'.* Instead of eating the same thing day-in and day-out, plan to have only a couple of 'strict days' a week; three or four 'moderate' days and a 'cheat day' *where you eat whatever you like!* This variation gives your body mixed signals, never giving it the opportunity to kick into its 'primitive survival mechanism', that stores fat at the slightest hint of famine.

A regular nutrition plan for fat loss should be for life, so this will prevent binging and craving and should make it a lot easier to stick at. When you reduce your food portion sizes, you will need to increase your protein intake by an extra 20%, to maintain your muscle mass and keep your metabolism in a high gear. Protein takes a while to digest and by staying in your system for a longer period, it provides your muscles with a steady stream of amino acids, maintaining your muscle mass and keeping your fat burning furnace stoked! Eating healthily doesn't have to be about avoiding the 'naughty' foods; it is about eating *lots of good food and ensuring you have a good balance of nutrients.*

On the whole home cooked meals using fresh ingredients are preferable to ready meals and why not try to finish the meal with a piece of fruit instead of a stodgy pudding!

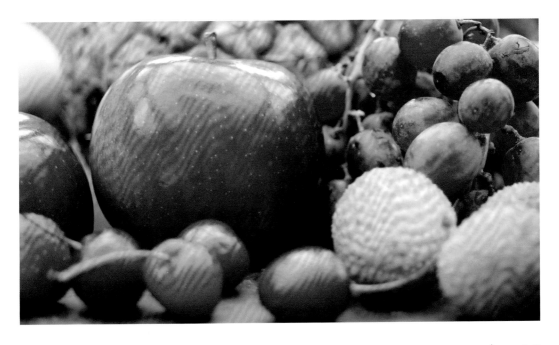

SECTION 2 - SEATED EXERCISES

A PROGRAMME OF DAILY SEATED EXERCISES
THAT YOU CAN TRY AT HOME TO IMPROVE YOUR
QUALITY OF LIFE

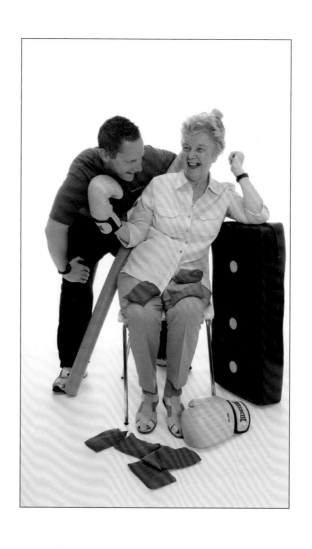

THESE MOVEMENTS WILL
PHYSICALLY AND MENTALLY
PREPARE YOUR BODY FOR THE
EXERCISES TO FOLLOW

POSTURE IN THE CHAIR

First of all find an armless chair and sit tall, spine into the back of the chair, feet and knees hip distance apart, and lengthen the neck. If your feet don't touch the floor, find a large book to place under your feet. Keep the tummy muscles nice and tight but don't hold your breath.

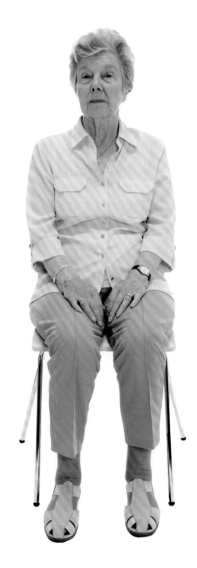

TIP   Always check body posture before starting any new exercise

ARM SWINGS

Place your arms by your side and gently swing them backwards and forwards, keeping a nice continuous and smooth swinging action (no jerky movements).

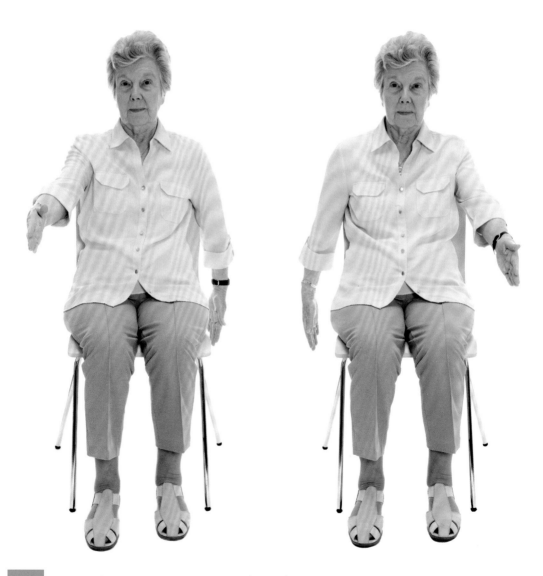

TIP Keep the movement smooth and continuous

SHOULDER ROLLS

Arms by your side take the shoulders up to the ears, backwards and then well down, in a slow circular movement.

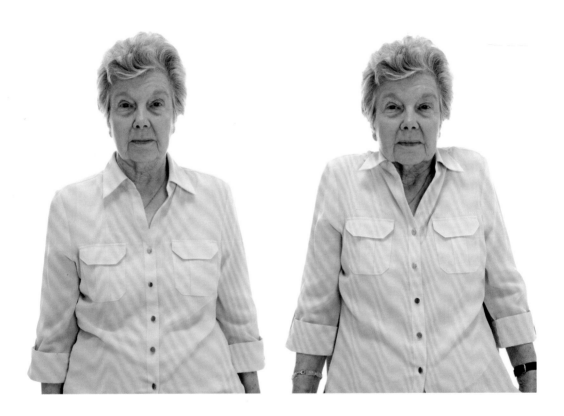

Continue this movement until you feel a warm feeling across your shoulders or you have achieved 10 shoulder rolls.

TIP Keep the motion continuous with no jerky movements

WRIST ROTATIONS

Raise one hand off your lap and rotate in a big circular movement for 10 seconds, then do the same with the other hand.

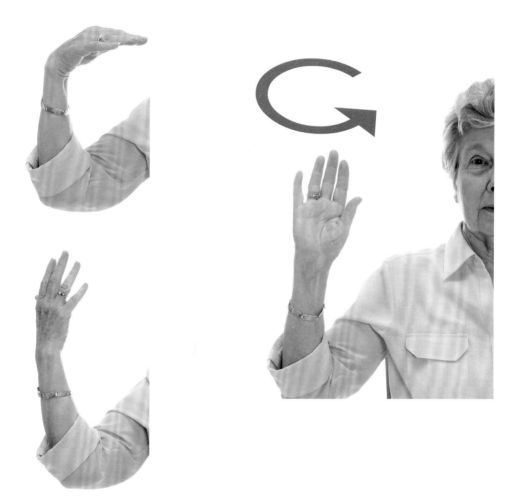

TIP This is great exercise to perform daily to keep your wrists supple

ELBOW RAISES

Place your arms by your side with a 90° angle at the elbow, so your forearms are parallel to the floor. Maintaining this position, raise your elbows and forearms together out to the side to your fullest range of movement, but no higher than shoulder height. When you have reached your fullest range of movement, slowly return to the start position and repeat 8 times.

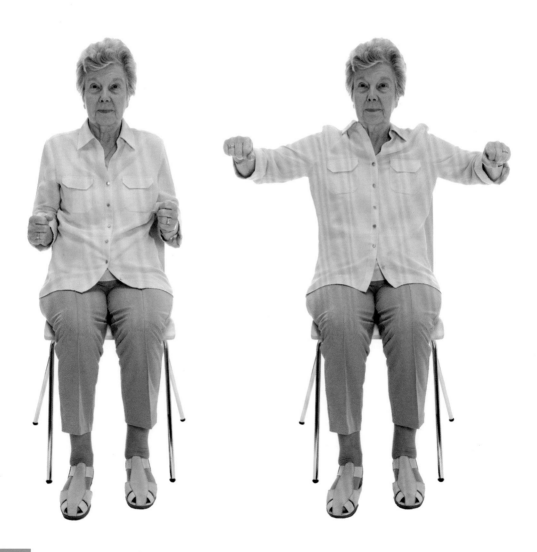

TIP Keep your chest lifted to maintain a neutral spine

UPPER BODY TWIST

Move your spine from the back of the chair, keep your feet flat on the floor and lengthen your spine, cross your arms and when you are ready, twist the upper body to one side keeping your head looking in the same direction as you are twisting (just like in the picture). When you have reached your fullest range of movement, return back to the middle, pause, and then twist to the other side, keeping the movement slow and controlled, and finally return to the start position.

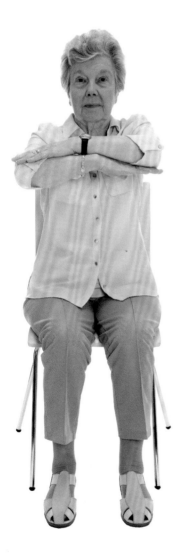
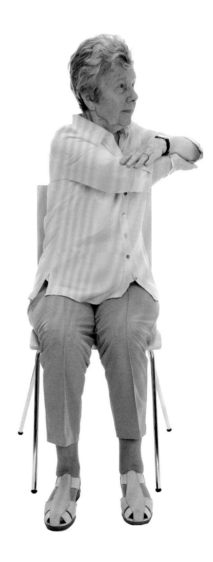

KNEE RAISES

Sit in the chair and re-check your posture. Sit tall with the spine in the back of the chair. Place both hands under the upper part of one leg and raise the foot off the floor - don't raise the leg too high - then lower the foot back down. Repeat 5 times on each leg.

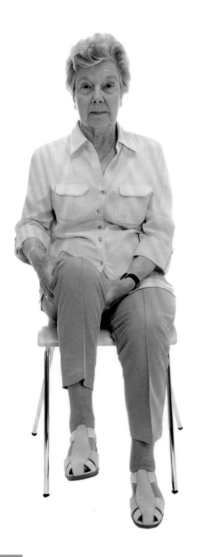
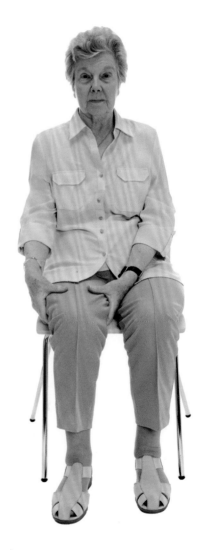

TIP Do not raise your leg to high if you have had a hip replacement

ANKLE ROTATION

Raise one foot in front of you so that it is off the floor and rotate the foot in one direction for 10 seconds.

Now complete the same movement but in the other direction for 10 seconds.

Repeat this action again with the other leg, remembering to rotate the foot in both directions.

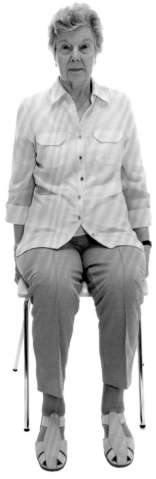 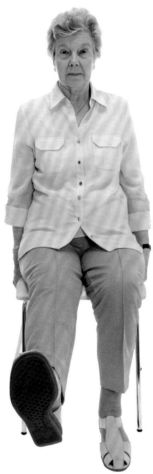

To challenge your coordination, try the same exercise with both feet together in one direction and then repeat in the other direction. Finally, rotate one foot in one direction and the other foot in the other direction.

HAND CLAPS

Starting slowly, clap your hands and slap your thighs continuously so that you feel your shoulder muscles begin to feel warm and your heart rate increases.

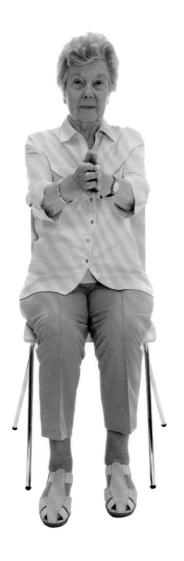
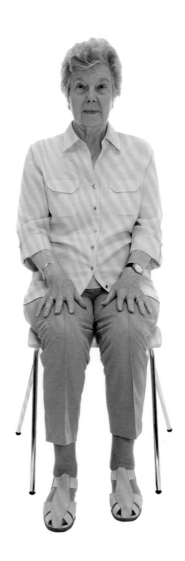

MARCHING

Keeping your arms by your side gently start to march your feet, this time you should find the tops of your legs and hips begin to feel warm. Depending on your fitness levels this could take a few seconds or a few minutes.

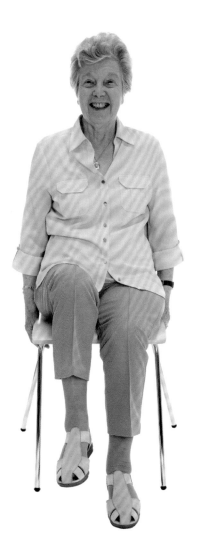 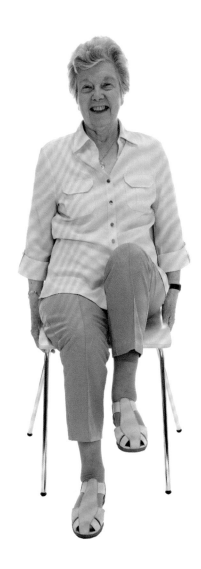

TIP This is great exercise to perform daily to keep your hips supple

SIDE STRETCH

Link your fingers together and press your hands towards the ceiling. Stretch your arms up as high as you can and hold the stretch for 10 seconds. Then unlink your fingers and push your arms out to the side to allow your arms to return to their natural position by your sides.

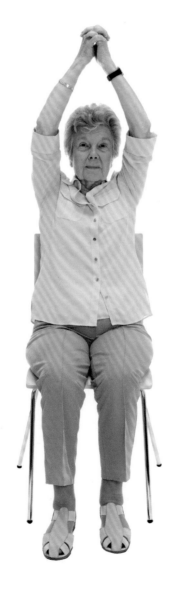

TIP Avoid holding your breathe with any stretches

HAMSTRING STRETCH

Move towards the edge of your chair then straighten one leg out in front of you with the heel on the floor pulling the toes back towards your body. You should feel a stretch running down the back of the straight leg, hold the stretch for 10 seconds - then repeat with the other leg.

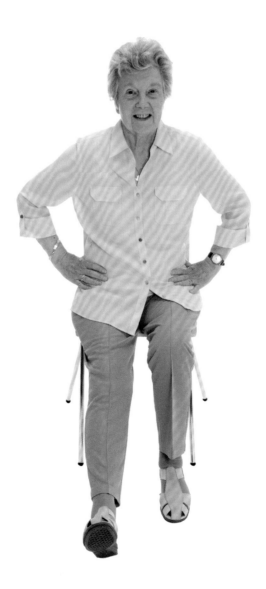

FINGER STRETCH

Place both hands out in front of you and spread your fingers apart like a star fish, hold the stretch for 10 seconds.

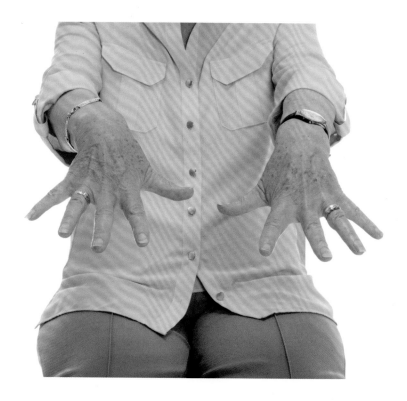

TIP Try wriggling your fingers before this stretch

TRICEP STRETCH

Put a bend in your arm and with the opposite hand hold on to your elbow Raise the elbow up towards the ceiling whilst keeping the bend in the arm that you are stretching and hold it for 10 seconds - then repeat with the other arm.

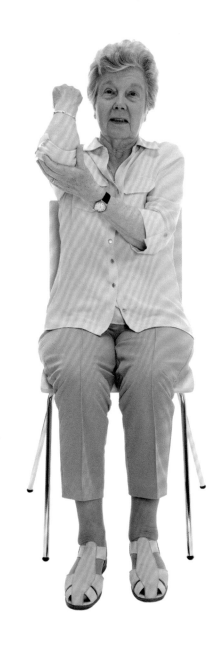

CALF STRETCH

Lift one leg off the floor straight out in front of you, then pull your toes towards your body to feel a stretch in the back of the lower leg, hold for 10 seconds - then repeat with the other leg.

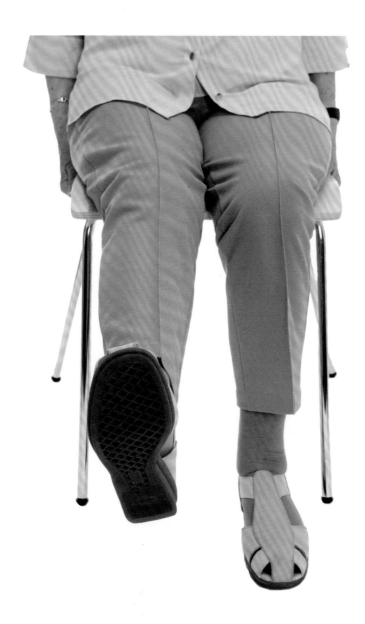

THESE EXERCISES WILL IMPROVE
YOUR GENERAL HEALTH AND
FITNESS

ARM SWINGS

Caution: If you're breathing so fast that you are unable to hold a conversation, slowly reduce your effort in the exercise you are doing.

Sit tall, spine into the back of the chair, feet and knees hip distance apart and lengthen the neck. Place your arms by your side and gently swing them backwards and forwards just like a soldier. Keep the movement continual and try not to make the movement jerky. Keep your arms swinging until they begin to feel warm around the shoulder area - this could be a few seconds for some people or a few minutes for others, depending on your fitness level!

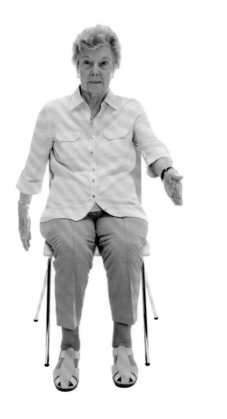 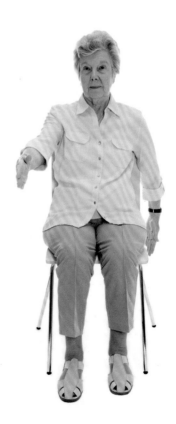

TIP	Try to keep each movement continual and exert yourself so that you are feeling slightly puffed

MARCHING

Keeping your arms by your side gently start to march your feet this time you should find the tops of your legs and hips begin to feel warm. Again depending on your fitness levels this could take a few seconds or a few minutes.

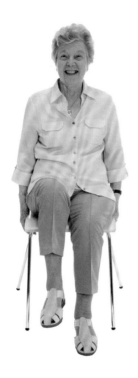 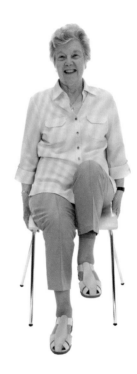

Progression: Repeat the whole sequence and if you are still not finding that you are getting slightly puffed and warm, increase the time for which you do the marching. **(Remember you only need to get to a level where you feel slightly puffed)**. As your fitness improves you can introduce 'speed intervals', where you will 'pitter-patter' your feet as fast as you can for 10 seconds, rest, and then when ready add another speed interval and so on. This is a great, safe and fun way of challenging your cardiovascular system.

TIP   Always check body posture before starting any new exercise

ARM ROLLS

Keeping your chest lifted to lengthen the spine, lift your arms and roll your hands around each other in front of you at shoulder height. Continue until your arms begin to feel heavy. Rest, and then restart the movement rolling the hands in the opposite direction for the same amount of time.

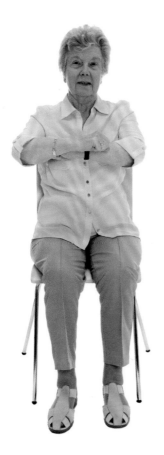 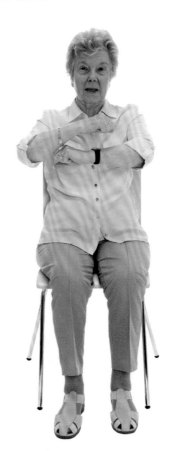

Progression: This movement can be introduced whilst marching at the same time and, for an added challenge, try marching the legs as fast as you can while rolling the hands forward as slowly as you can!

TIP Always work at a comfortable pace

THE FOLLOWING STRENGTH EXERCISES WILL IMPROVE YOUR BODY POSTURE AND MAKE EVERYDAY TASKS EASIER

BICEP CURLS

Push your spine into the back of the chair, keep feet and knees hip distance apart and lengthen the neck, keeping the tummy muscles nice and tight - **but _don't_ hold your breath!**

Clench your fists up and place them on your lap, keeping your elbows down, then bend your elbows to raise your hands towards your chest and then lower back to the start position – repeat this 8 times.

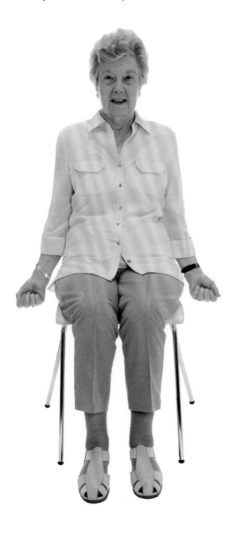
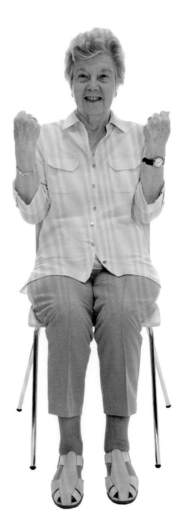

TRICEP EXTENSIONS

Bend your right arm so your right hand is touching your right shoulder. With the other hand under the elbow, raise the elbow in front of you level with the chest. Now you are in the 'start' position, extend the arm out in front of you till it is straight and then with control return to the start position – repeat 8 times with each arm.

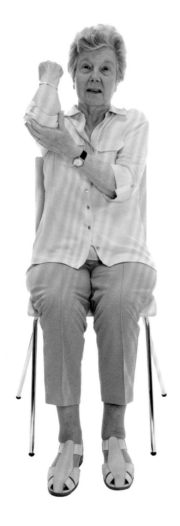 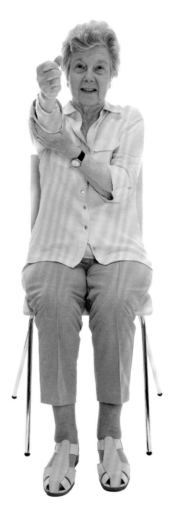

TIP Always work to your fullest range of movement

ELBOW RAISES

Place your arms by your side with a 90° angle at the elbow, so your forearms are parallel to the floor. Maintaining this position, raise your elbows and forearms together out to the side to your fullest range of movement, but no higher than shoulder height. When you have reached your fullest range of movement, slowly return to the start position and repeat 8 times.

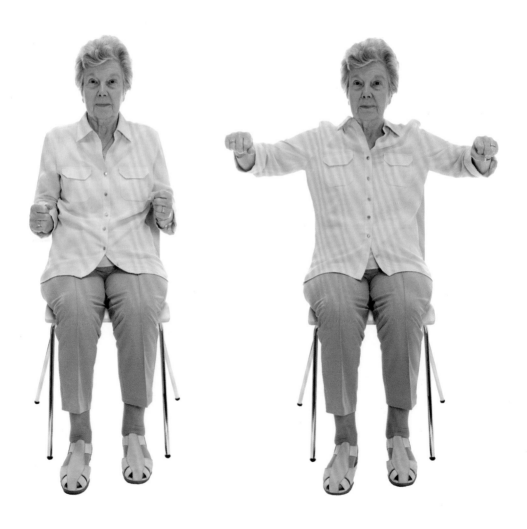

TIP Keep your chest lifted to maintain a neutral spine

ROWING

Imagine you are in a little rowing boat holding on to imaginary oars. Start rowing your arms backwards and forwards. Repeat the movement 8 times.

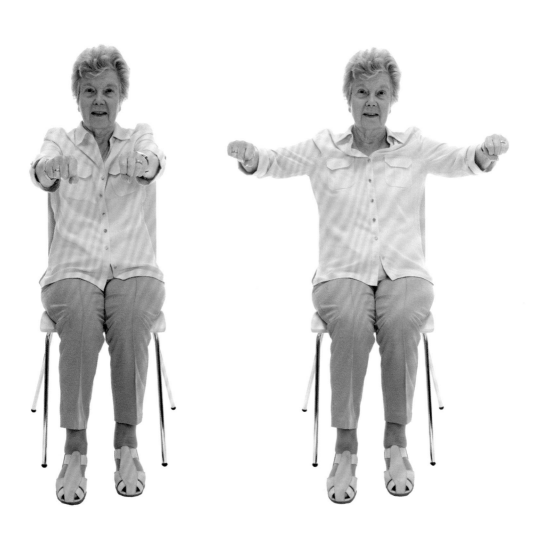

SINGLE LEG EXTENSION

Place both feet on the floor in front of you. Extend one foot and leg in front and pull the toes up towards you. When the leg is fully straightened, slowly return the foot back to the floor, allowing the heel to gently touch the floor. Repeat the movement 8 times. Once you have completed the exercise with one leg repeat with the other.

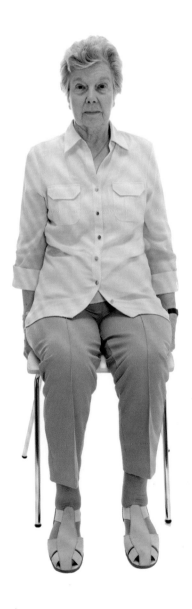
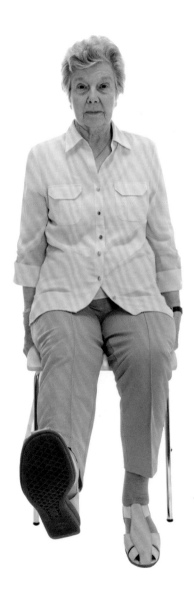

DOUBLE LEG EXTENSION

Place both feet on the floor in front of you. Extend both feet and legs in front and pull the toes up towards you. When the legs are fully straightened, slowly return the feet back to the floor, allowing the heels to gently touch the floor. Repeat the movement 8 times.

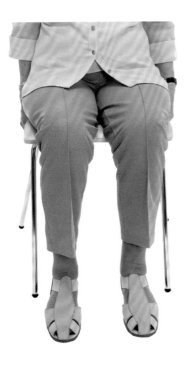
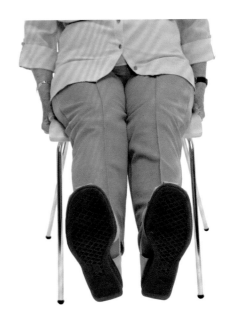

TIP Keep your spine pressed against the back of the chair

UP AND DOWN OUT OF CHAIR

Caution: This exercise is not suitable for everyone and should be performed with care!

Place your chair an arm's length away from a secure, steady table and after sitting down, shuffle forward so that your legs are away from the chair. Then, place the palms of your hands lightly on the table in front of you and your feet hip distance apart on the floor *(see the picture for the correct position before going any further)*. From here, lifting upwards from your head, stand up. To sit down, shuffle back so that your legs are touching the chair *(feel the chair with the back of your legs)*, slowly bend your knees and lower onto the chair. Now all you need to do is repeat this another 4 times!

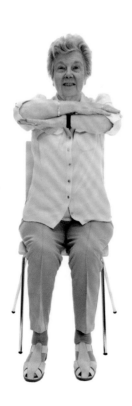 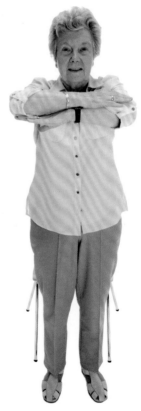

NOTE For purposes of clarity the table is not shown

THESE STRETCHES WILL IMPROVE YOUR FLEXIBILITY AND ALLOW YOU TO COOL DOWN GENTLY

MARCHING

Keeping your arms by your side gently start to march your feet, you should find the tops of your legs and hips begin to feel warm. Depending on your fitness levels this could take a few seconds or a few minutes.

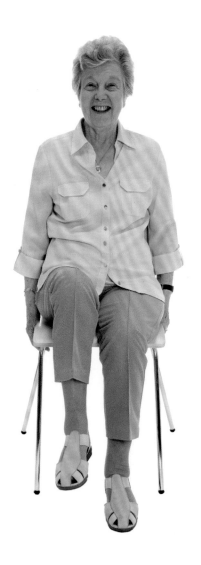 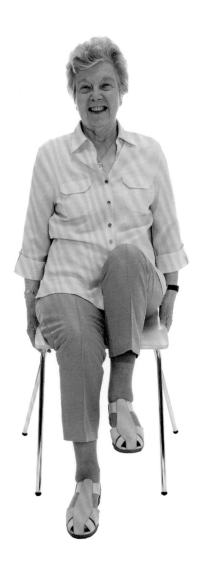

ARM SWINGS

Place your arms by your side and gently swing them backwards and forwards, keeping a nice continuous and smooth swinging action (no jerky movements).

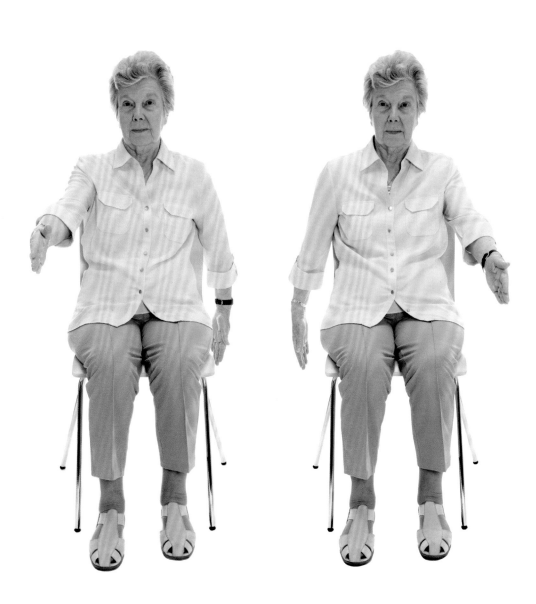

SHOULDER ROLLS

Arms by your side take the shoulders up to the ears, backwards and then well down, in a slow circular movement.

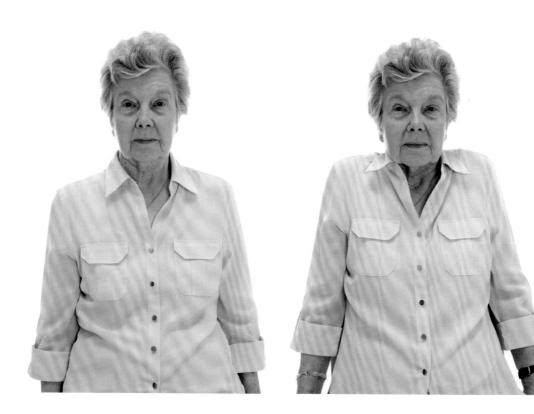

Continue this movement until you feel a warm feeling across your shoulders or you have achieved 10 shoulder rolls.

WRIST ROTATIONS

Raise one hand off your lap and rotate in a big circular movement for 10 seconds, then do the same with the other hand.

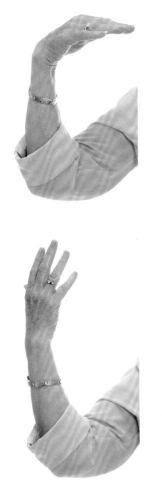

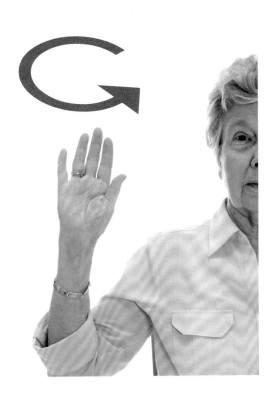

ANKLE ROTATION

Raise one foot in front of you so that it is off the floor and rotate the foot in one direction for 10 seconds.

Now complete the same movement but in the other direction for 10 seconds.

Repeat this action again with the other leg, remembering to rotate the foot in both directions.

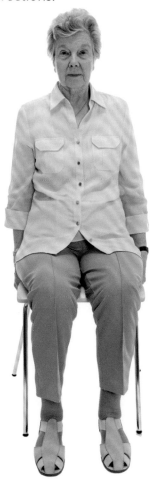 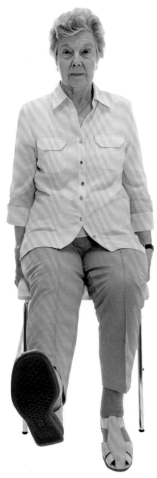

To challenge your coordination, try the same exercise with both feet together in one direction and then repeat in the other direction. Finally, rotate one foot in one direction and the other foot in the other direction.

TRICEP STRETCH

Put a bend in your arm and with the opposite hand hold on to your elbow. Raise the elbow up towards the ceiling whilst keeping the bend in the arm that you are stretching and hold it for 15 - 20 seconds - then repeat with the other arm.

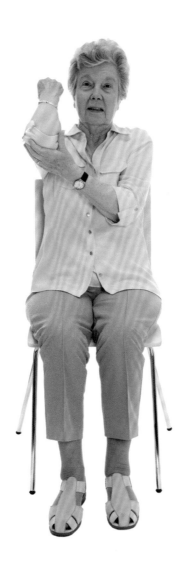

SIDE STRETCH

Link your fingers together and press your hands towards the ceiling. Stretch your arms up as high as you can and hold the stretch for 15 - 20 seconds. Then unlink your fingers and push your arms out to the side to allow you arms to return to their natural position by your sides.

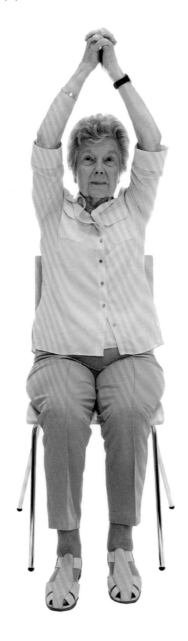

HAMSTRING STRETCH

Move towards the edge of your chair then straighten one leg out in front of you with the heel on the floor pulling the toes back towards your body. You should feel a stretch running down the back of the straight leg, hold the stretch for 15 - 20 seconds - then repeat with the other leg.

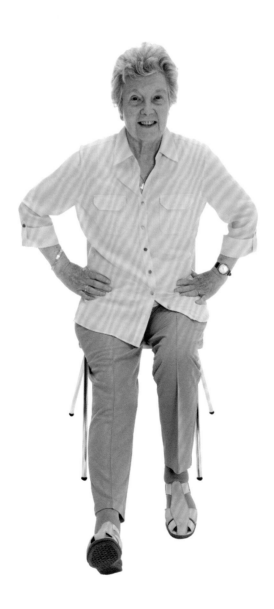

FINGER STRETCH

Place both hands out in front of you and spread your fingers apart like a star fish, hold the stretch for 15 - 20 seconds.

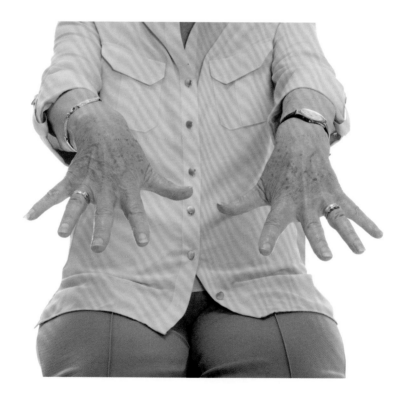

CALF STRETCH

Lift one leg off the floor straight out in front of you, then pull your toes towards your body to feel a stretch in the back of the lower leg, hold for 15 - 20 seconds - then repeat with the other leg.

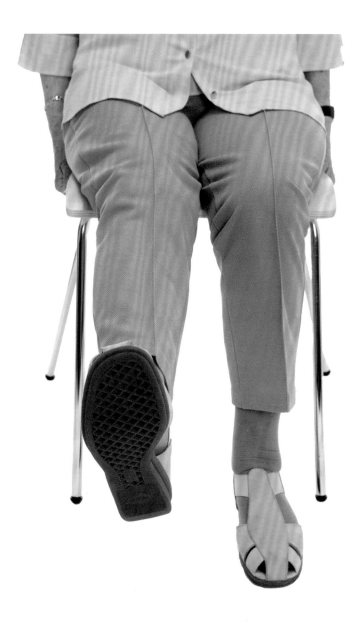

CONCLUSION

I hope that you have found this book useful and that it has shown you how to introduce physical activity into your lifestyle.

Please continue to practise the seated exercises on a regular basis and you will find that this will contribute to a better quality of life. Many of the clients that I work with have reached their short term and long term goals giving them a new lease of life.

Now that you understand that physical activity is not just structured exercise you can find many other daily activities to achieve your 30 minutes of moderate intensity exercise on most days of the week.

My final piece of advice to you is to find as many opportunities as you can and try to socialise with different age groups! Getting out into the fresh air each day is beneficial: you feel less stressed and looking around you can have a calming influence. In most areas a range of health walks are run by local councils and further information about other types of walks can be obtained from libraries or Information Centres or are listed on a variety of websites. Dancing is an excellent form of exercise and is a great way to make new friends! Why not join a singing group, or an art class or book circle to keep your mind active too! If you can't find one – why not start your own?

Above all enjoy life and find time to laugh and smile with your family and friends and make the most of the natural world.

ACKNOWLEDGEMENTS

Special thanks are due to John Price who photographed many of the pictures in this book and who helped me put together the design of this book.

I would also like to thank Hettie Williamson who kindly donated her time to model for the seated exercise photographs and who has been a friend and supporter of the work that I do.

Thanks are due to the following people for helping with the editing, proof reading and general advice on producing this book, Julie Chandler, Bob Rawlinson and Tricia Moxey.

Diana Powley for inspiring and supporting me in achieving one of my long term goals of writing this book and for writing the page on "Relaxation".

For the people featured in this book, namely Hettie Williamson, my daughter, Amelia Hogg, my wife's grand parents Maureen and Bernie Giardelli, Julie and Glyn Cooper with Mike Perry in the allotments, Dorothy with her window box and Tricia Moxey pegging out the washing.